100 Questions and Answers About People Who Stutter

A Listener's Guide

Michigan State University School of Journalism in cooperation with the Department of Communicative Sciences and Disorders

Front Edge Publishing

For more information and further discussion, visit

biasbusterguides.com

ISBN: 978-1-64180-252-9

Version 1.0

Cover design by Rick Nease

RickNeaseArt.com

Published by

Front Edge Publishing

44932 Ford Road, No. 234

Canton, MI

Front Edge Publishing books are available for discount quantity purchases for events, corporate use and small groups. For more information, contact Front Edge Publishing at info@FrontEdgePublishing.com.

Contents

Acknowledgments

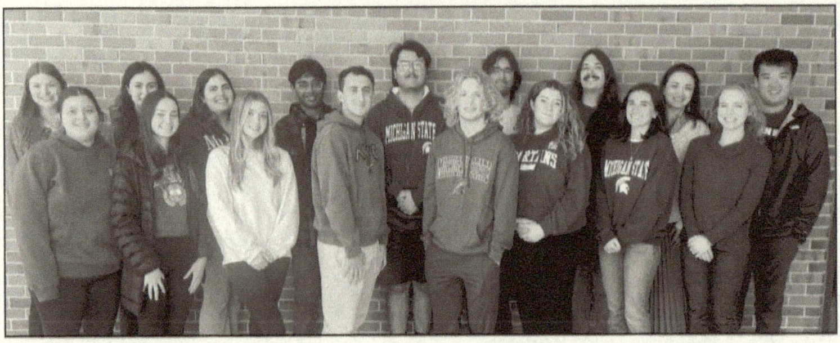

These are the Michigan State students who created this guide. Front row from left: Alison Garon, Sadie Carlson, Sophia Gorman, Nicolas Fardella, Maxwell Waier, Natalie McLaughlin, Mia Thistlethwaite and Megan Arney. Top row from left: Lindsey Van Hekken, Bailey Marino, Kelsey Mae Grzymski, Shreshta Sinha, Joshua E.K. Kresnak, Ayushya Gautam, James Peetz, Jia Bin, Travis Yang. Also: Gwendolyn Urbain. Van Hekken shot and produced the video interviews that appear in the guide.

This publication was greatly informed by people who stutter and more than a dozen researchers and speech-language pathologists. They generously contributed their experience and expertise. Professor J. Scott Yaruss and Sharon Emery were chief among them. They encouraged the class from before we began, visited to speak, reviewed drafts and wrote some of the introductory material that follows. They elevated this guide.

Other contributors:

Jia Bin, M.A., a doctoral student at Michigan State University, was a consultant in this course. Bin earned an undergraduate degree in English language and literature at Chongqing Normal University in China and a master's degree in secondary education at Oakland University. She earned a master's degree in Communicative Sciences and Disorders at Michigan State University. Bin has been a language teacher (English and Mandarin Chinese) and has taught in China, the United Kingdom, and the United States. Bin is motivated to bring people together by her journey as a person who stutters and an inter-cultural communicator.

Megan Arney, Ph.D., CCC-SLP, was also a consultant in this course while a doctoral student at Michigan State University. She is an assistant professor at the University of Wisconsin-Stevens Point, where she earned her master's degree in speech-language pathology. Arney has been a speech-language pathologist in school, hospital and clinical settings with all ages. Her research interests include stuttering and its impact on a person's life.

Angelica Bernabe is a person who stutters from Peru and she is director of the Specialized Center for Stuttering (Centro Especializado en Tartamudez). She earned her degree in clinical psychology in Peru and her M.A. in speech-language pathology at Michigan State University. She is a Ph.D. student at Florida State University. In 2022, Bernabe won the Clinician Award from the World Organization of Stuttering and Cluttering for helping people throughout Central and South America.

Patrick Briley, Ph.D., is an associate professor in the Department of Communication Sciences and Disorders at East Carolina University. He focuses on conceptualizing stuttering and understanding what contributes to the overall impact of stuttering.

Shelley B. Brundage, Ph.D., CCC-SLP, BCS-SCF, is a fellow of the American Speech-Language-Hearing Association and a professor of speech, language and hearing sciences at George Washington University. Her research interests include the use of virtual reality in clinical education for stuttering.

Caryn Herring, Ph.D., CCC-SLP, F-ASHA, is a person who stutters and a speech-language pathologist. She is executive director of Friends: The National Association of Young People Who Stutter, a nonprofit support organization. Her research focuses on desensitization, reducing the adverse impact of stuttering, and improving accessibility for individuals who stutter.

Robert Quesal, Ph.D., CCC-SLP, F-ASHA, was a professor emeritus of communication sciences and disorders at Western Illinois University and a person who stutters. An ASHA fellow, he served as associate coordinator and newsletter editor for the American Speech-Language-Hearing Association Special Interest Division for Fluency Disorders.

Lee Reeves, D.V.M., a retired veterinarian, has been a member of the American Speech-Language-Hearing Association Specialty Board for Fluency Disorders and the ASHA Council for Clinical Competence. He was chairman of the board of directors for the National Stuttering Association and is CFO for Stuttering Therapy Resources, Inc. Quote: "I have been stuttering for about 70 years, and I am getting pretty good at it."

Naomi H. Rodgers, Ph.D., CCC-SLP, is an assistant professor of communication sciences and disorders and director of the Stuttering Lab at the University of Iowa. She focuses on cognitive, emotional and social factors in developmental stuttering.

John Tetnowski, Ph.D., CCC-SLP, BCS-SCF, F-ASHA, holds an endowed chair in Speech Pathology at Oklahoma State University and is an ASHA fellow. He has more than 25 years of clinical experience and has published more than 85 manuscripts on fluency disorders and research methods.

Seth E. Tichenor, CCC-SLP, is an assistant professor and program director with the Stuttering Clinic in the Department of Speech-Language Pathology at Duquesne University in Pennsylvania. Interests include differences in stuttering experiences, how moments of stuttering occur and how adversity develops.

Bridget Walsh, Ph.D., CCC-SLP, is an associate professor and undergraduate program director in Communicative Sciences and Disorders at Michigan State University. She researches the development of stuttering and its adverse impact on children.

Barry Yeoman was interviewed for this project and connected us to many other experts. He then helped us improve our questions and read a draft. Yeoman has won dozens of awards as a multimedia investigative reporter. Yeoman teaches journalism at Wake Forest University and Duke University. He has a B.A. in journalism from New York University and was a Knight-Wallace fellow at the University of Michigan.

Thanks to **Jon Whiting**, digital storytelling professor of practice in the MSU School of Journalism, who advised on the videos.

Several people appear in the videos and met the student authors at a panel and in a stuttering support group. They include **Kristen May**, **Trevor Moran** and **David Potts**, Ph.D.

Two leaders in MSU's College of Communication Arts and Sciences supported this project. They are **Tim P. Vos**, Ph.D., School of Journalism professor and director, and **Dimitar Deliyski**, Ph.D., MSU Foundation Professor and chair of the university's Department of Communicative Sciences and Disorders.

Foreword

By Dr. J. Scott Yaruss

Stuttering is a widely misunderstood experience that affects the lives of roughly 80 million people worldwide. People who stutter face discrimination in the form of limitations in educational opportunities, reduced earning and job prospects, hurtful comments and bullying by others, difficulty in social and romantic life, and more.

Stuttering is often portrayed in the media as a sign of weakness, insecurity, or a lack of intelligence. Public perceptions of stuttering and of those who stutter are overwhelmingly negative, and it is not uncommon to hear people make disparaging comments about those who stutter or to imitate stuttering for comedic or dramatic effect.

It is not surprising that all this societal stigma has a highly detrimental effect on the lives of people who stutter. People who stutter are more likely to experience social anxiety, to withdraw from social interactions, to try to hide their stuttering from others, and even to harbor suicidal thoughts.

This book seeks to reduce the negative beliefs and biases that society holds about stuttering. Using a format of 100 questions and answers, it provides key facts about what stuttering is, explains why people stutter, and presents more helpful ways that people can interact with individuals who stutter. Here is a taste of what you will learn:

- Stuttering is different from the types of disruptions that all people experience in their speech from time to time. Everyone has moments when they aren't sure what to say. People who stutter have those too, but they also have moments when they know exactly what they want to say but are unable to say it the way they want or when they want.
- To a listener, the moment of stuttering can sound like a repetition of sounds, a sound that is stretched out longer than expected, or a time when no sounds come out at all. These moments of stuttering can be accompanied by tension or struggle as the person tries to force their words out.
- To a speaker, the moment of stuttering feels like a "loss of control" of the speech mechanism. People who stutter say that they feel "stuck" when talking, and when they feel this, they do things to try to get unstuck.
- Stuttering is caused by neurological differences that are largely believed to be genetic in origin. It is not a psychological problem or something that people learn from others. It arises due to differences in the brain.
- Stuttering typically starts during early childhood, at a time when speech and language skills are developing rapidly. Children do not pick it up from listening to others stutter, and it is not caused by a traumatic event. It is also not caused by any mistake that parents might make in raising their child.
- People who stutter are not doing anything wrong when they stutter. They are simply speaking in a way that is consistent with their neurology. Recognizing that stuttering is not their fault helps to reduce some of the blame that people often feel for speaking differently from other people.

- Stuttering is variable: the amount of stuttering that people experience in one situation or at one time is not the same as the amount of stuttering that they experience in another situation or at another time. This is not because they are lazy or not trying hard enough; it is simply the nature of stuttering.
- Many people who stutter can learn skills that help them say what they want to say more easily, but not all people want or need to do this. Such changes, if desired, can be found through speech therapy conducted by a skilled speech-language pathologist or through stuttering self-help or support organizations.
- It is generally not considered helpful for listeners to speak for people who stutter, to fill in words, or to avoid talking to people who stutter. People who stutter want to speak for themselves, just like everyone else does.
- As a society, we can help people who stutter by becoming more accepting and understanding of stuttering and by recognizing that the person who stutters can benefit from additional time to say what they want to say. In fact, the most helpful thing that a listener can do is to simply wait patiently while a person who stutters is talking, giving them the time they need to express themselves.

The authors and editors of this book seek to create a world in which people who stutter do not face hardships imposed by societal stigma … a world in which they can be appreciated and valued for *what they say* rather than how they say it. By reading this book, you are taking an important step in bringing that dream to reality.

Thank you for taking the time to learn about stuttering and about people who stutter, and for contributing to a world that is supportive of different ways of speaking.

J. Scott Yaruss, Ph.D., CCC-SLP, BCS-SCF, F-ASHA, H-ASHA, is a professor of Communicative Sciences and Disorders at Michigan State University, where his research is funded by both the National Institutes of Health and the National Science Foundation.

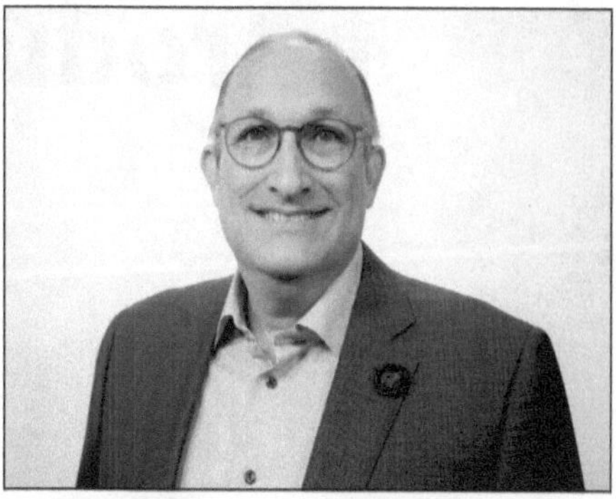

He has been a practicing speech-language pathologist specializing in stuttering for more than 30 years. He has published more than 140 peer-reviewed papers, as well as more than 400 other books, papers, chapters, and articles. He has also given more than 850 invited presentations on stuttering, as well as more than 275 reviewed presentations. He is also the president of Stuttering Therapy Resources, Inc., a specialty publishing company dedicated to helping speech-language pathologists help people who stutter.

Introduction

By Sharon Emery

I'm a "communications-impaired" woman who has made a career in communications. I know, go figure.

I have been a newspaper reporter and editor, a university instructor, a public relations consultant, an author … and a person who stutters. Since forever. Sometimes severely. Still, even now.

The way I've come to survive stuttering — when I was young the struggle was painfully real — and finally to thrive, is to think about stuttering as my accent. It's simply the way I talk. Everyone has their own speaking style; this is mine.

Of course, that approach requires listeners to get with the program. In a world that values fast-talkers and fluency, they have to learn to listen differently and patiently. A tall order, I know.

My advice to listeners: Get used to it and you'll be fine. And I will be, too, since you won't be judging my speech.

That's where this book comes in.

Speakers who stutter, here's a comprehensive, thoroughly researched look at what you're facing. You likely already know a lot about stuttering, but you'll find important information you don't.

Listeners, buckle up. You likely will have to learn how to listen better. The good news: helpful tips are included.

Difficult speech is, undeniably, difficult … both to listen to and, especially, to produce.

It took me decades to learn that I have a public speaking voice. It just happens to include a stutter. I have even given speeches about how to give speeches, to fluent speakers who think they can't give speeches. It's a crazy world we live in.

But every time I speak in public — be it at a conference of some bigwigs or the local fast-food drive-through — somebody's mind gets blown. And that's a good thing.

Whenever you speak to a person who stutters, they're recalibrating their speech to ensure they get their message across. Likewise, listeners should be recalibrating their listening to make sure they're fully participating in the conversation.

Ideally the mechanics of stuttered speech and the mechanics of adaptive listening will ensure that we're communicating. That's what this book hopes to facilitate.

The potential is awesome: The extent to which confident speakers and attentive listeners can adapt our various abilities during a single conversation can be our contribution to making the world a better place. No kidding.

There are a million little ignorances in the world, some of which are yours to fix. Please blow them up when you can. This book can show you how.

Be you speaker or listener:
Be unashamed.
Be unafraid.
Good luck!

Sharon Emery
June 2025

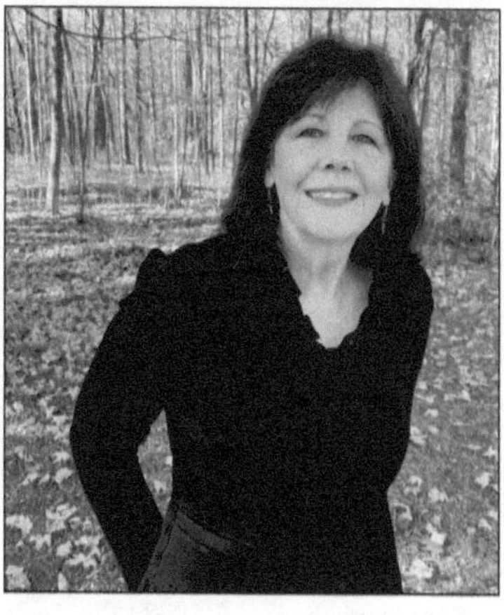

Preface

By Joe Grimm

Listen patiently.

That is the key message in this guide.

Wherever you go in the world, about 1 percent of the population stutters. This guide is for the other 99 percent of us.

Work on this guide was started by a journalism class at Michigan State University in the fall of 2024. That October, "International Stuttering Awareness" month declared a motto. It was, "People who stutter have the unique opportunity to teach the world to listen."

That made sense to us. If there is a problem, it is in the way most of us listen rather than the way 1 percent of us speak. Maybe efforts to cure stuttering would be better spent on curing the way people listen. So that is our goal.

If we can better understand stuttering, how it works, how it feels and how we can live with it, we can narrow the fluency gap. If we can learn to listen better to all people, well, then we will really have something.

These 100 questions come from asking what people who stutter want readers of this book to know. That knowledge became our guide to better listening.

We regularly welcomed people who stutter into the class to speak. We interviewed individuals. We attended stuttering support groups. One group included a pre-law student, a supply chain management major, a neurology student and a doctoral candidate. They were asked, "What would you like people to know about you?" Their answer: "That we are intelligent."

How sad. These people obviously are smart. But because many listeners fixate on how people speak rather than on what they are saying, we miss the message.

We can do better. We can listen. If listeners work as hard as people who stutter, we can understand.

Joe Grimm
Michigan State University
School of Journalism
Series founder and editor

People Who Stutter

1 What is stuttering?

People who stutter have a difference in speech production in which they sometimes feel "stuck" when producing words and sounds. Some people "block" on certain sounds. They simply can't get it out without considerable effort. Others may repeat sounds. Speakers who stutter often have little control over disfluencies. They may physically struggle to produce words, and listeners may see gestures or movements that people who stutter make as they talk. How often and how much people stutter varies with the situation, the complexity of what they are saying and the type of conversation. People who stutter may experience fear or anxiety about speaking, and this can affect all aspects of the person's life.

2 What are disfluencies?

Disfluencies are not stuttering. They are breaks in the smooth or fluent flow of speech. Examples include repeating phrases or using interjections such as "um." Disfluencies typically indicate that a person is thinking about what to say. Disfluencies may also occur when people change their mind and revise what they are saying (for example, "I want — I need that"). People are not judged for disfluencies, but they are judged for stuttering.

3 What is the distinction between stuttering and other types of disfluencies?

Everyone has occasional moments of disfluency as they plan what they want to say. When people stutter, however, they are not simply planning what they want to say. Stuttering involves a sensation of being unable to move forward in speaking, even when the person does know what they want to say. That moment of feeling stuck can be very unpleasant for people who stutter. It is unlike what people who do not stutter experience.

4 Is it OK to call people "stutterers?"

Many people who stutter prefer to use "person-first" language. That is, "person who stutters." This puts the person in front of the disorder rather than highlighting the condition. They don't want to be defined by just one aspect of themselves. Some other people who stutter are reclaiming the label "stutterer," though it was once used to put them down. These individuals proudly self-identify and refer to themselves as "stutterers," seeking to counteract social stigma. When referring to a group, either term is usually understood to include all people who stutter. When referring to an individual, it is better to ask their preferred term if the relationship allows you to talk directly about their stuttering.

5 What types of stuttering are there?

While there are many types of disfluencies, there are two primary types of stuttering conditions.

1. **Developmental stuttering** typically begins between the ages of 2 ½ and 4. About 5-8 percent of children go through a period of stuttering. In 75 to 80 percent of cases, stuttering stops before the child reaches the school-age years. For the other 20 to 25 percent, stuttering continues into adulthood. This type of stuttering affects three or four times as many men as women. Approximately 1 percent of adults around the world stutter, including roughly three million in the United States. This type of stuttering is a neurodevelopmental condition that arises from subtle differences in brain regions involved in language planning and speech production.
2. **Acquired stuttering** can develop at any age, though its usual onset is in adulthood. It is usually caused by a stroke or other type of brain injury, psychological trauma or other unknown factors. The person's experience of this kind of stuttering varies depending on the nature of the injury.

Patterns

6 Is stuttering occasional or constant?

For people who stutter, the condition is always present, but they do not typically stutter on every word or sentence. Stuttering is highly variable, occurring more or less in some situations or at some times than others. This may make it seem as if people are in control of their speech. Sometimes, people can tell when they are about to stutter, but other times stuttering may take them by surprise. They are always mindful of their condition.

7 Is stuttering predictable?

One of the most frustrating qualities of stuttering is that it is not predictable. It changes with circumstances. Sometimes people can sense that they are more likely to stutter, but sometimes they cannot. Some factors make stuttering more or less likely to occur. Stuttering frequency and duration can be high or low, even in the same day, depending on self-image, anxiety, eagerness, excitement, weariness and worry. All can impact the way stutterers speak. These factors differ from person to person, and even within the same person over time.

8 Are there different kinds of disfluencies?

There are many types of disfluencies. For example, there are repetitions of sounds or syllables ("li-li-like this"). There are repetitions of whole words or phrases ("like-like-like this"). Some disfluencies are produced by all people (including interjections such as "um"). Other disfluencies tend to be produced more by people who stutter (such as blocks, where no sound at all comes out).

9 Are "um" and "like" disfluencies?

Interjections, also known as filler words, are common in the speech of all people, both those who stutter and those who do not. Interjections include words such as "um," "uh" and "like." They typically reflect a moment when a person is thinking of what they want to say. People who stutter also use interjections when they are thinking about what they want to say. Or they may use them in an attempt to avoid a moment of stuttering.

10 Are certain words or sounds more difficult?

Many people who stutter say some words or sounds are more difficult than others. The specific words or sounds differ between people and may change over time. Some have trouble with words that begin with vowels; others struggle with words that start with specific consonants. Furthermore, the purpose of words can affect whether a person finds a word to be difficult. For example, some people find nouns and verbs to be more difficult.

11 Are stuttering and stammering different?

Stuttering and stammering mean the same thing. Stuttering is the preferred term in North America and Australia. Stammering is preferred in the United Kingdom, Ireland and India, according to the International Stuttering Association.

12 Is there gender bias in treatment or research?

Most research has focused on male stutterers, according to a study published in a journal of the American Speech-Language-Hearing Association. Perhaps fewer women are studied because fewer of them stutter. More research could reveal important differences in how female and male stutterers are treated socially or at work.

13 Is culture a factor in stuttering acceptance?

Culture does not cause stuttering, but there are cultural differences in how listeners perceive and react to it. Some groups have less knowledge about or tolerance for stuttering. This can influence the experience of the person who stutters. Ignorance, intolerance or a lack of trained speech professionals can mean less acceptance and more shaming.

14 How do people with stuttering succeed?

People who stutter have achieved great success in many fields. Yet even the most accomplished say that stuttering can intrude and impede their ability to communicate. It can shake their confidence and frustrate them. This frustration comes both from the difficulty of speaking and from the way that others react to stuttering. This leads many people who stutter to develop secondary behaviors in response to these reactions.

Behaviors

15 What are secondary behaviors?

People who stutter may exhibit various movements as they struggle to speak. Behaviors may include facial expressions, gestures or body movements. These are also called "secondary characteristics." They typically develop over time as people cope with reactions to their stuttering.

16 Should I look away when a person stutters?

Many people who stutter feel that maintaining eye contact normalizes the stutter to both speaker and listener as part of the conversation. Some people who stutter say maintaining eye contact helps them hold other people's attention and feel more in control. Listeners should maintain natural eye contact when someone stutters and be patient. Looking away can signal disinterest. In general, watch the other person for cues and follow their lead.

17 Is stuttering related to Tourette syndrome?

No. The two may co-exist, but they are distinct conditions. People who stutter might also have Tourette syndrome, but one does not cause the other, according to the Stuttering Foundation. People with Tourette syndrome may exhibit motor or verbal tics including speaking disfluencies. These uncontrollable behaviors may be due to differences in the levels of a chemical neurotransmitter. Individuals with Tourette syndrome might produce more non-stuttered behaviors, such as clicks, whistles and unrelated remarks. These are not the same types of behaviors as stuttering or as stutterers' secondary characteristics.

Better Listening

18 What do supportive listeners do?

Good listeners are patient and attentive. This may be difficult for listeners who are uncomfortable with stuttered speech. If stuttering makes you uncomfortable, maintain eye contact and use active listening skills. These include nodding your head to confirm understanding. Interrupting with suggestions such as "slow down," "relax," or "take a breath" are condescending and rude. People who stutter do not appreciate this simplistic advice. Do not finish a person's sentences or try to guess the words they're saying. Stutterers deserve the dignity of speaking in their own unique voices.

19 What happens when listeners "fill in the blanks?"

While the intent may be to help, supplying words interrupts people. It implies their voice and thoughts are not valued. However, in some cases people who stutter might not mind if others finish their sentences. Listen and watch to understand your conversation partner's preferences. Being patient and giving people room to express themselves creates a more supportive, respectful conversation.

20 What is helpful eye contact?

Maintaining a natural connection with someone who stutters means neither continuous staring nor looking away. It takes a mix to show engagement and attention and to help the speaker feel at ease. Eye contact can help even during moments of stuttering. Just wait patiently. Listeners who look away when someone stutters can create awkwardness for both the speaker and the listener. Remember that standards for eye contact can differ by culture and might have nothing to do with stuttering. Standards can vary based on expectations and societal norms. Watch the speaker's preferences for eye contact and try to mirror them.

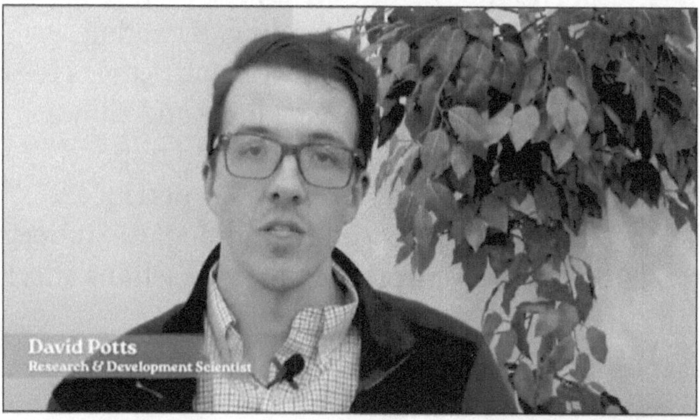

Hear how you can be better at listening to people who stutter. It is not difficult. It takes kindness, patience and practice. Follow the link or scan the QR code to watch: youtu.be/odH21Fgv5cM

21 Is it better to just ignore stuttering?

Focus on listening to what a speaker is saying rather than how they are saying it. If you sense that someone who stutters is frustrated with the conversation, ask how you can make it more productive. Be open to the speaker's advice. Even if you make a mistake, keep talking with them. Most speakers will appreciate your efforts to be a good listener.

22 Is it rude to ask people who stutter to repeat themselves?

No. We do this with everyone we want to understand. It's more respectful to ask for clarification than to guess. Guessing can lead to misunderstanding. By asking clarifying questions, we show that we value people's ideas and want to understand them. Ask kindly and allow people the uninterrupted time they need to respond. People who stutter can anticipate it and experience it physically, emotionally and with their thoughts. Stuttering can feel like a loss of control, and others' reactions affect that.

23 What does stuttering feel like?

Many people who stutter describe stuttering as a sensation of feeling "stuck." They also describe it as a sense of "losing control" of their speech. They know what they want to say, but it does not come out as planned. This loss of control is often frustrating, and it can lead to anxiety and embarrassment. This makes it harder for people to say what they want.

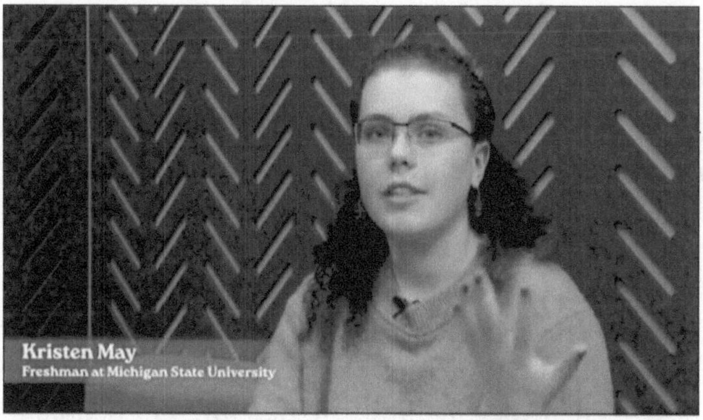

What does stuttering feel like? Follow the link or scan the QR code to watch: youtu.be/8cNN6lfKu6E

24 Is stuttering a hidden condition?

Stuttering is noticeable only when people talk. There are no visible impairments, no equipment such as crutches or canes, and nothing different about the way people move about or work or play. Having a stutter is not always immediately obvious. People may not stutter in all situations, and some limit talking to avoid having their stutter noticed and judged. Thus, stuttering can be hidden or concealed.

25 Is stuttering a disorder or a disability?

Stuttering is classified as a "fluency disorder" under the broader heading of communication disorders. Stuttering is not a mental issue, a psychological problem or a learning disability. The Americans with Disabilities Act of 1990 protects people who have "a physical or mental impairment that substantially limits one or more major life activities." That can include people who stutter, depending on how their stuttering limits them. Different people who stutter have different perceptions and experiences. These can change throughout a person's life. Some people face stuttering limitations that can be classified as a disability; others do not. Allow individuals who stutter to decide for themselves if they are facing a disability rather than automatically labeling them without their input.

26 What is wrong with having a disability?

Some people who stutter object to the label. To view stuttering as a disability is to categorize people as disabled. This can reflect negatively on the people who live with it. Others freely say they have a disability and work through it, taking pride in how they overcome and achieve. It is important not to diminish or discount people who stutter and to privilege those who do not.

Coping

27 What can people who stutter do about it?

Many people who stutter seek out support groups or speech therapy. In groups, they can meet and talk with others who stutter. In therapy, they can learn ways of speaking more easily and handling stuttering more effectively. Support groups and therapy can help people learn to reduce the challenges they face due to stuttering.

28 How do people try to reduce stuttering?

People use several techniques to try to reduce the frequency or intensity of stuttering moments. Many techniques have been developed to help people speak more easily so that they can say what they want to say, even when they stutter. Some techniques involve changes to how people speak. Some involve helping people handle moments of stuttering as they occur. Putting pauses between phrases can allow time for framing and bringing out statements.

29 How do support groups work?

These are groups of people who stutter and who gather to talk about ideas and experiences. The groups can help people feel more comfortable talking and facing their shared communication differences. People report that participating in a self-help or support group reduces the sense of judgment and isolation that they experience. The groups help people view their stuttering in a more neutral or even positive fashion. One reason for this is the solidarity and camaraderie with others. Knowing you are not alone in facing a challenge can be uplifting. The groups talk about advocacy and coping or are just social. There is a growing number of stuttering associations, camps and online support groups. Self-help groups are led by peers rather than professionals. The National Stuttering Association maintains a list of local meeting groups at WeStutter.org/chapters.

30 Do word substitutions help?

People who find that specific words seem to trigger stuttering moments may choose different ones, but this is not considered helpful. Pressure to anticipate stuttering and quickly swap words can be exhausting. Swaps cause people to use words other than the ones they really want to say.

31 How do people try to conceal or mask stuttering?

Some people avoid situations where they might have to talk. This can isolate them socially or limit their verbal participation at school or work. These are ways of being a "covert stutterer." Trying to hide the fact that they speak differently from others can put a lot of pressure on people. If stuttering were better understood and accepted, this would not be necessary

32 What does speech therapy do?

Therapy is individualized and follows a plan to improve various aspects of a person's communication. In therapy, individuals may learn to adapt speech patterns that support the forward flow of speech. Comprehensive speech therapy addresses cognitive, emotional and social reactions to stuttering.

33 Can reading aloud help reduce stuttering?

Some people who stutter find that they stutter less while reading aloud. However, this is not always the case. Reading is sometimes used in therapy, but just to practice speaking skills.

34 What does it mean to stutter openly?

Some people who stutter don't try to hide it. This is called stuttering freely or "just" stuttering. Many speakers find that when they don't try to hide their stuttering, listeners come to accept it. They also can relate to others more deeply.

Roots

35 Does stress cause stuttering?

Stress does not cause stuttering. Stress can raise the amount of tension that people experience and increase the frequency of stuttering. This is like the way that anxiety can disrupt speech or other activities in anyone. All people might produce more disfluencies when they feel anxious. Often, stress arises due to the difficulties inherent in different speaking situations and to the reactions that listeners have to stuttering. This can make it harder for people who stutter to say what they want.

36 Is stuttering genetic?

Stuttering often runs in families, suggesting that genes are a contributing factor. Also, comparative studies of identical and fraternal twins support a genetic component. Stuttering is not purely genetic, however. Research has shown that genetics is not the sole factor behind stuttering.

37 Are there degrees of stuttering intensity?

Some people stutter more than others. Some stutter so rarely that listeners have difficulty detecting it. At different hours, individuals may stutter more or less, depending on circumstances. These differing degrees of stuttering can be seen in how much physical tension or struggle they exhibit, and how much they stutter or try to hide it.

38 Does the social environment affect stuttering?

Different factors can increase or decrease stuttering, and the effects vary among people. Some individuals stutter more when talking to large groups of people, though some stutter less before large groups. Some people stutter more when talking to authority figures, while others stutter less. Pressure for fast talk, such as ordering at a drive-through, can make stuttering more likely. We are still learning about all the ways and reasons that affect stuttering.

39 Is stuttering contagious?

One cannot "catch" stuttering by being around people who stutter. It is not learned from others, either. People who do not stutter but who feel they did after talking with someone who does are just briefly more conscious of their own disfluencies. They could even be imitating what they hear, but this does not last.

Physiology

40 Where does stuttering originate?

Stuttering arises from factors related to planning what one wants to say and then saying it. These abilities are determined by neurological structures and functions. Factors related to planning what to say and how to say it may contribute to the loss of control. Stuttering may also involve differences in coordinating muscles that control breathing, producing one's voice and articulating speech sounds.

41 Which part of the brain handles speech production?

Speech production involves several key brain areas, such as Broca's area for planning speech movements and Wernicke's area for language formulation and comprehension. Both are critical for speaking. The primary motor cortex controls the muscles involved in speaking. The basal ganglia and cerebellum coordinate these motor movements. The auditory cortex processes the feedback that allows speech to be self-corrected during production. Studies show that stuttering is associated with differences in the structure and function of several parts of the brain. Different parts regulate motor function, emotions and relaying information.

42 Are language formulation and speech production the same?

They are separate but must work together. Language formulation is the process of planning what one wants to say and how one wants to say it. Speech production is the process of saying the sounds and words that have been planned. To formulate language, the brain must access the right words, assemble sentences and process language at the neural level. To produce speech, one must coordinate breathing, producing voice, and moving the mouth to create sounds. Difficulties in any of these processes can disrupt speech, and these disruptions can increase with the complexity of the task.

43 Do people who stutter process speech and language differently?

Yes, there are differences. Somehow, the process is disrupted in people who stutter. This disruption could be occurring in one or more brain areas related to language and speech or in the connections among them.

Neurology

44 Is stuttering a sign of lower intellect?

There is no difference in intellect or intelligence between people who stutter and those who do not. Although people who stutter can have difficulty getting words out, they know how to speak and what they want to say.

45 Can a brain injury cause stuttering?

Most of this book refers to a type of stuttering sometimes known as "developmental" stuttering. This type of stuttering is not associated with brain injury but rather differences related to how the brain develops. Another type, acquired stuttering, can be caused by psychological or physical trauma. Physical trauma could include a head injury or stroke affecting parts of the brain associated with language planning and speech production. The duration of this kind of stuttering varies depending on the injury.

46 Would brain imaging hold a key to stuttering?

Neuroimaging techniques such as magnetic resonance imaging, magnetoencephalography, electroencephalography and functional near-infrared spectroscopy have been used to study brain activity in people who stutter. These studies reveal differences in the structure and function of regions involved in language planning and speech production.

Speech Therapy

47 Does speech therapy help?

Many people who stutter benefit from speech therapy. The professionals best qualified to help are speech-language pathologists, called SLPs or "speech therapists." People may seek therapy to help them speak more easily or to address challenges associated with stuttering. If parents are concerned about a child's speech, they and the child should meet with a speech-language pathologist to determine if therapy is recommended.

48 How does speech therapy work?

Speech therapy can help people handle stuttering so that it is less of a problem in their lives. For very young children, therapy may focus on reducing the chances that they will continue stuttering into adulthood. School-age children, adolescents and adults may learn skills for speaking and communicating more easily. This may include learning to handle moments of stuttering effectively, learning to reduce anxiety related to speaking and becoming more open about stuttering. Over time, this can help them say what they want to say more easily.

49 What do speech-language pathologists do?

Speech-language pathologists diagnose and treat issues related to articulation, fluency, voice and resonance, language, cognition, hearing, swallowing, social communication and alternative forms of communication. Certified SLPs hold the "Certificate of Clinical Competence in Speech-Language Pathology," or CCC-SLP, issued by the American Speech-Language-Hearing Association, or ASHA. SLPs are also licensed by state professional licensing boards. SLPs work with people from birth through the end of life. They work in various settings including hospitals, schools, skilled nursing facilities and private practices.

50 What training do speech therapists receive?

To be certified to work with people who stutter, speech-language pathologists complete several steps of training. First, they must earn an undergraduate degree, often in the field of communication sciences and disorders. With the correct prerequisite classes, students completing any major can pursue a career in speech-language pathology. Students must then earn a master's degree in speech-language pathology. This is typically a 1½- to 2-year program. These programs provide training in human communication and disorders. After the master's degree, candidates complete a clinical fellowship. This is supervised by a certified speech-language pathologist. Successful completion of the clinical fellowship leads to certification.

51 Are there clinicians specifically for stuttering?

Certified SLPs can continue their academic and clinical education to receive board certification as specialists in stuttering. This is managed by the American Board of Stuttering, Cluttering and Fluency Disorders. Certification requires many hours of training and clinical work with children and adults who stutter. Clinicians seeking specialty certification must also demonstrate advanced skills.

52 What is cluttering?

This is a different kind of disorder in which words come in bursts and unevenly, with unexpected pauses. Cluttering can include jumbled words, incomplete sentences and mid-stream corrections. Whereas people who stutter are very aware of how their speech sounds, people who clutter might seem to be unaware. Cluttering may occur with or without stuttering.

53 Does singing reduce stuttering?

Some people who stutter can sing with little or no apparent stuttering. The reasons for this are still being debated, but the brain is used in different ways for singing and speaking. In any case, singing is not a useful component of therapy for stuttering.

54 What are major speech-therapy approaches?

People who stutter can learn various speaking skills to reduce the appearance or intensity of stuttering. Although these skills are relatively easy to learn, they are difficult to use and maintain over the long term. Many people who stutter benefit from therapy that focuses on reducing their negative reactions to stuttering. This may be accomplished through cognitive therapies. Some examples are cognitive-behavioral therapy (CBT) or acceptance and commitment therapy (ACT). These approaches may be used with therapy focused on changing people's speech. Importantly, therapy should be individualized and tailored to each speaker's preferences, needs and goals.

55 Are there enough speech-language pathologists?

There are not enough SLPs who specialize in stuttering to meet demand. According to CareerStaff Unlimited, SLPs who work in schools are not getting paid enough for their caseloads. Therapist shortages and high caseloads are signs that schools need to spend more in this area. According to the U.S. Bureau of Labor Statistics, the number of SLPs grew 18 percent from 2022 to 2023. According to the National Institutes of Health, more clinical education opportunities for stuttering are needed. Fewer than 1 percent of SLPs say they have enough training to help people who stutter.

56 Can stuttering be cured?

Many young children who stutter stop while they are still in the preschool years. Individuals who continue to stutter beyond age 6 or 7 are likely to continue stuttering in some fashion throughout their lives. There is no cure for stuttering in school-age children, teens, or adults. Still, effective therapy can help them speak and communicate more easily and cope with stuttering more effectively. This can help ensure that stuttering does not negatively impact their lives.

57 Should stuttering be cured?

That depends on whether you see stuttering as a problem or as a part of human diversity. People who stutter often have negative views about their stuttering and themselves due to social interactions. If people who stutter were not judged negatively, then it would be less of an issue for them. There would be less of a desire for a cure.

58 What is stuttering pride?

The stuttering pride movement seeks to remove negative stereotypes about stuttering. It opposes mocking, teasing and shaming. The pride movement affirms all forms of speaking "as beautiful in all its voluntary and involuntary utterances." In the introduction to "Stammering Pride and Prejudice: Difference not Defect," the authors write, "Stammering is often seen as a joke, and it is taken for granted in our society that fluency is better than stammering. But … this is not necessarily true. Stammering can benefit both people who stammer and society if we let it."

Social Impacts

59 How does stuttering harm self-esteem?

We live in a fluent, fast-talking world, so some people who stutter feel pressure to try to fit in and talk like other people. This can hurt self-esteem, and the negative influences can begin early. Studies show that children and adolescents who stutter are bullied more often than those who do not. Intervention by parents and educators can help. However, negative social reactions to stuttering are the real problem.

60 Is social anxiety linked to stuttering?

Some studies indicate that people who stutter experience social anxiety more than people who do not. The anxiety that people who stutter may experience goes beyond nervousness or being shy. It can cause people to talk less and reduce social interactions to avoid microaggressions.

61 What are stuttering microaggressions?

Microaggressions are comments or actions that can be hurtful for people, even when they are not intended that way. Consider the messages behind these phrases: "I hardly noticed your stutter." "You sounded normal that time." "Slow down." "It's not so bad to stutter." Individuals who stutter hear all these statements. Though people may be well-meaning when they say such things, the result is greater isolation and shame for people who stutter. Microaggressive actions include looking away when someone stutters, interrupting to speak for them, or making motions to hurry them along. "Micro" applies to the reality that, even though microaggressions seem small, they pile up over time and are cumulatively harmful.

62 Do people who stutter isolate themselves?

Many do, and this is one reason why many therapists recommend group therapy. A report by Mayo Clinic suggests that some people who stutter isolate themselves to avoid embarrassment and negative reactions. They may avoid speaking situations, as well as social, school and work interactions. If you know someone who stutters, try to talk with them and include them in activities. This helps bust the stigma.

63 Do people stutter when no one is around?

People who stutter when talking with other people are much less likely to stutter while alone. Studies going back decades have shown this. Researchers reason that people who stutter do not worry about being judged when they are alone.

64 Does stuttering make people introverts?

The combination of low self-esteem, isolation and social anxiety can make people who stutter become more introverted. However, like all people, people who stutter have different personalities. Some may indeed be introverts. Others may be more extroverts or ambiverts, a balance of the two. Studies have found that extroverted people who stutter have a more positive attitude toward communication. In contrast, people who stutter may be shy about speaking. That does not make them introverts.

65 Can stuttering affect dating?

Experiences with dating for all people vary. While some people who stutter say they experience difficulties, others say they do not. Some may avoid talking to someone they like out of fear of rejection. A study in the Journal of Fluency Disorders found that young adults perceive people who stutter to be less attractive. The study also found that people who do not stutter were less likely to want a romantic relationship with someone who does.

66 Why does stuttering make some listeners feel uncomfortable?

Listeners who have little exposure to stuttering may not know how to react. This may make them uncomfortable. Understanding that stuttering is just a different way of speaking can help both listeners and speakers. The National Stuttering Association has a simple recommendation: Be patient. Wait for people to finish their sentences before responding, and do not interject.

Families

67 Does home life cause stuttering?

Home life does not cause stuttering, but it can influence how a person experiences stuttering. Children who already stutter and who are pressured to speak in a particular way might stutter more. However, this is not the cause of stuttering.

68 How can parents best help young children who stutter?

Parents can do a lot to help their children who stutter. The ways they can help depend upon the child's age. Roughly 5 to 8 percent of very young children stutter. Approximately 75 to 80 percent of them will stop stuttering before their school-age years. Parents who are concerned about their child's stuttering should consult a speech-language pathologist for guidance about whether an evaluation or treatment is recommended. This is true even for very young children who have just started stuttering. In therapy, parents and other caregivers can learn about how to support their child's communication at home and in other settings.

69 What can parents do for older children?

As children age, the strategies that help them may change. Older children can learn skills that make it easier for them to say what they want to say. Like all interactions with people who stutter, parents should avoid interrupting their children or finishing their sentences. By focusing on what the child is saying, they can show that what the child wants to say is important. As children grow, they may face new challenges, such as bullying. Parents can work with speech-language pathologists, teachers and others in the child's environment to ensure that the child is supported.

70 How can families help children build self-confidence?

Family dynamics, support and communication shape how people who stutter view themselves and their speech. Open discussions about stuttering can help normalize it. This reduces feelings of shame or embarrassment. Family members can emphasize that stuttering doesn't define the child. By focusing on the child's message rather than their apparent fluency, parents can help children be more confident in their speech.

71 Can home life hurt children who stutter?

Although families do not cause stuttering, they can react to stuttering in ways that are less helpful. One way this might happen is if a family member bullies the child about stuttering. Even well-meaning "jokes" can cause emotional harm, leading to lower self-esteem and fear of communicating.

School

72 How does stuttering affect learning?

Stuttering does not inhibit the ability to learn. However, the anxiety that may accompany stuttering can make it hard for students to engage at school. Children who stutter may experience difficulties with reading out loud, asking and answering questions and public speaking. Some students try to avoid these activities. This can reduce learning opportunities and harm participation grades.

73 How can educators help students who stutter?

Teachers can create a safe learning environment for students who stutter. They can encourage a relaxed atmosphere in which all students have time to speak. Educators should immediately intervene in any bullying and minimize interruptions when a stuttering student is speaking. They can also foster an open dialogue with the student and work with the student's speech-language pathologist to meet their unique needs.

74 How does bullying affect students who stutter?

Bullies target students who stutter. Studies in several countries show that students who stutter are bullied more than others. Furthermore, anxiety and speaking difficulties experienced by children who stutter can make it harder for them to stand up to bullies. This can increase the occurrence and impact of bullying. Fortunately, there is much that children can do through therapy to diminish both the occurrence and the impact of stuttering.

75 Does stuttering impede learning to read and write?

Stuttering is about speaking, not intelligence or comprehension. Studies have shown that stuttering does not affect a student's ability to learn how to read and write. Timed oral reading tests may be difficult for students who stutter because of the time pressure. However, there is no difference between silent reading ability in students who stutter and those who do not. As a group, people who stutter can comprehend written words as well as other people.

76 Do people who speak more than one language stutter in all of them?

In general, people who stutter and who speak more than one language will stutter in all of them. Still, there may be language differences in how they experience stuttering. For example, some people may stutter more in their native language than in other languages they have learned. Others may stutter more in their newer languages. These differences can change over time, like other variables in the stuttering experience. It is important to recognize that being multilingual does not make stuttering more likely. It was once thought that multilingual people were more likely to stutter. Research has shown that this is not true.

77 Are students eligible for school accommodations?

U.S. schools are required to accommodate students who meet federal disability criteria. Students qualify if a mental or physical condition "substantially limits one or more major life activities." In U.S. schools, accommodations may be part of the student's Individualized Education Plan (IEP). These could be speech therapy, extra time on presentations or exemptions from classroom activities involving speaking aloud.

78 What other support is available for students who stutter?

Elementary and secondary school children who stutter but who do not require special education and an IEP may get a 504 plan. This can include quiet spaces for testing and the option to present information in audio or print. They can also get outlines of lessons.

Employment

79 How does stuttering affect job prospects?

Studies show that 70 percent of people who stutter believe their condition hurts their chances of being hired. Some may not apply for jobs that require oral communication because they doubt they can do the job well or because of their fear of speaking. Job interviews can be stressful for anyone but especially for people who stutter. Many employers are unfamiliar with stuttering. They may believe that stuttering will hinder the individual's ability to excel in a job. However, people who stutter can and do succeed in all kinds of jobs every day.

80 Do people who stutter get paid less?

Studies have shown that people who stutter tend to get paid less. A 2018 study published in the Journal of Speech, Language, and Hearing Research found that people who stutter earned $7,000 less per year than those who did not. Different variables, including education level and hours, played a role in that. For women, the gender pay gap compounds stuttering salary deficits.

81 Do people who stutter have difficulty in phone or video conference calls?

Many people who stutter report feeling stress during conference calls and Zoom sessions. They may be concerned that they will be ignored or talked over if they experience a block. Video calls can help with this, but it can also introduce new challenges. People may be uncomfortable watching themselves stutter or being magnified on the screen in front of others. People can turn off self-view or their cameras but may still feel disadvantaged.

82 What accommodations can help workers who stutter?

Employers are required to make reasonable accommodations to help people succeed in the workplace. One accommodation is allowing a person to communicate via email when appropriate, rather than requiring them to use the telephone. Another is educating employees in the work setting about stuttering and encouraging patient, respectful listening. Not everyone who stutters will need or ask for accommodations. Employers who adapt these habits make for an inviting, high-functioning workplace where everyone can fully contribute.

83 Do people who stutter experience discrimination at work?

Many say they experience discrimination by colleagues and employers. In an article for the Society of Human Resource Management, CEO Jahanzaib Ansari described discrimination he faced due to his stutter. Stuttering is covered under the Americans with Disabilities Act, so people who stutter have legal protection from discrimination. People who face job discrimination can file a complaint with the federal Equal Employment Opportunity Commission. However, it is difficult to win job discrimination cases.

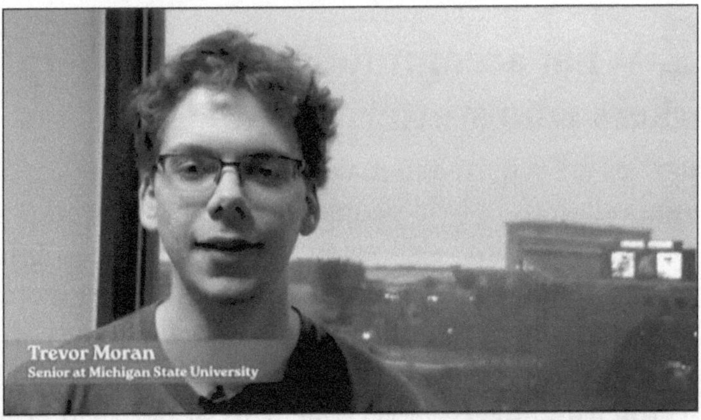

Stutter friendly workplaces or classrooms value people who stutter for what they say and don't judge them for how they say it. Two people explain. Follow the link or scan the QR code to watch: youtu.be/Zz-CAliPCBsWShwKESHzwlP

84 What characterizes a stutter-friendly workplace?

The first step is to hire qualified people despite their stuttering. Colleagues and supervisors can educate themselves about stuttering and learn to respectfully interact with people who stutter. It helps if the workplace culture values listening and discourages interrupting or aggressive interactions. The National Stuttering Association describes stutter-friendly workplaces as those in which people who stutter have readily available accommodations. The association maintains that making people who stutter feel valued goes a long way toward building an inclusive space.

85 Do people who stutter decline promotions?

Yes, many people who stutter experience insecurity at work. They may believe they are not competent enough to advance, or they may fear the speaking demands associated with more advanced positions.

86 Does stuttering affect advice on career paths?

An article in the Journal of Fluency Disorders confirmed occupational "role entrapment" for people who stutter. Advisers less often encourage people who stutter to pursue careers with higher perceived communication needs.

87 Does the Americans with Disabilities Act cover stuttering?

The ADA protects disabled and impaired workers from job discrimination and unfair treatment. The act requires employers to make reasonable accommodations so people can do their jobs effectively. Changes should not place "undue hardships" on employers. Changes should not cause significant difficulties when considering the employer's size and resources.

88 What qualifies stuttering as an ADA issue?

People must show how stuttering affects them at work. For workers who stutter, issues may arise from public speaking, telephone work, or fast-paced verbal exchanges. This could include the emotional and physical aspects of the stuttering and their perceptions of co-workers' reactions. Accommodations can vary from job to job and person to person.

89 What are reasonable accommodations?

People who stutter can be permitted to use a preferred method of communication, such as writing. That could mean using email instead of phone calls. Accommodations also could mean encouraging patient listening, allowing more time for responses in meetings and avoiding interruptions.

Technology

90 Does voice technology help people who stutter?

Currently, most voice technologies don't accommodate stuttering. Although speech recognition systems can help people who do not stutter, they can frustrate people who do. When some systems encounter pauses, they may think people have stopped talking. This issue and other challenges with voice technology are increasing as more devices use speech recognition. Examples include phones, digital mail, cars, even household appliances. Engineers and speech-hearing pathologists are searching for ways to improve the tools.

91 Does incorporating artificial intelligence help?

AI systems can increasingly understand spoken language, but stuttered speech still seems to stump computers. This is becoming more of a problem as AI systems handle more functions and people. For example, when AI is used in job interviews, applicants who stutter may be misunderstood or cut off. This can reduce the chances that they will get a job.

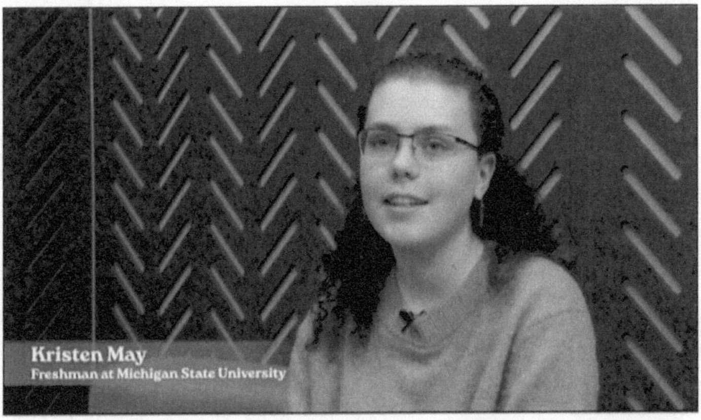

People who stutter and use Siri, Alexa, voice texting apps and other technologies do not get the same benefits from them as other people. In fact, voice-assist technology can be a barrier for people with speech disfluencies. Follow the link or scan the QR code to watch: youtube.com/watch?v=EPhFz-FDxr0

92 Can technology increase fluency?

Some systems have been designed to help people speak more fluently. For example, there is an effect known as "delayed auditory feedback." With this, people hear their own voice as they are speaking, but their voice is delayed by a fraction of a second. For reasons that are not well understood, people are less likely to stutter when speaking with delayed feedback. Unfortunately, the effectiveness of these approaches tends to decline. The search for technological aids that help people who stutter has been going on for years. Some aids have shown short-term benefits in apparent fluency, but evidence of long-lasting benefits is lacking.

93 Are there objections to technological solutions?

Although technology might help reduce apparent disfluencies, some people prefer not to surrender their own voice — including their stuttering — to seem fluent. According to The Stuttering Foundation, people who stutter do not wish for their speech to be replaced. They want to speak with their authentic voice.

94 Can teletherapy connect therapists to more people?

Teletherapy is connecting more people who stutter to speech-language pathologists. This technology can reach people who live in remote areas or who do not have access to a speech therapist. The American Institute for Stuttering reports that its clients rate teletherapy as effective as in-person sessions.

95 Is there a role for virtual reality?

Virtual reality headsets support research and therapy in a variety of ways. For example, researchers in several labs are partnering on simulations to understand how stuttering develops in young children. Other initiatives are creating real-life scenarios in the clinic. These help people practice what they learn in a variety of increasingly realistic situations.

Myth, Stigma and Stereotype

96 Are people who stutter stigmatized?

People who stutter experience two kinds of stigma: public and personal. Public stigmas involve negative societal judgments. People report being judged, condescended to, perceived as less intelligent, and overlooked in their achievements. Internalized negative feelings about one's own stuttering are called self-stigma.

97 What is the impact of social stigma?

Stuttering stigma can lead to emotional harm. Children who stutter can experience reduced confidence and self-esteem. They can become withdrawn, and their schoolwork can suffer. Adults who stutter report increased psychological issues such as depression and feelings of shame. Social impacts include isolation and loneliness. Employment and educational opportunities may be denied or avoided.

98 How does pop culture depict stuttering?

Movies, television and books depict stuttering in various ways. Many portrayals are negative and mocking. A few present a more realistic, positive image of stuttering. Erik Lamens, a filmmaker and president of the Belgian Stuttering Association, analyzed an international selection of 230 movies that had stuttering in them. He and his team categorized 31 percent of the movies as using stuttering to dramatize the story. A neutral approach, in which stuttering is simply present and not remarked upon, was in 27.5 percent of the movies. Stuttering was treated as a weakness in 16.4 percent of the movies and used as a joke or gimmick in 14.3 percent. Negative portrayals of stuttering contribute to societal stigma.

99 How do positive stuttering role models help?

Positive role models can help children and adults who stutter feel more confident. A study in the Canadian Journal of Speech-Language Pathology and Audiology showed that 85 percent of participants said having positive stuttering role models as children would have helped. Role models can inspire, offer coping strategies, create awareness and inclusive communities. Every person who stutters needs and wants different levels of support. Seeing people who are successful despite, or perhaps even because of their stuttering, can help. As civil rights activist Marian Wright Edelman noted, "You can't be what you can't see."

100 Who are some stuttering role models?

People who stutter are in every profession and walk of life. Leaders, executives, celebrities and people who are not famous stutter. Many of those people have experienced the same stigmas and feelings as others who stutter. Famous people who have stuttered include world leaders such as King George VI and President Joe Biden. Actors with a history of stuttering include Emily Blunt, James Earl Jones and Rowan Atkinson. Entertainers such as Elvis Presley and Bill Withers also stuttered. We can highlight famous people who stutter, but there are many more stuttering role models in our midst. These include individuals such as teachers and doctors, lawyers and plumbers, cab drivers and scientists. Everyday regular people who stutter and who have learned to cope with stuttering so that it does not stand in their way are examples of success stories.

Epilogue

Ultimately, this is the message that we want people to learn: even though stuttering can present challenges, people who stutter can live normal lives that are not negatively affected by stuttering. This is the ultimate goal of speech therapy, of self-help and support for people who stutter, and ultimately, of this book.

You can be part of the solution by listening patiently. By attending to what people are saying rather than how they are saying it, you will learn more from them and help all of us.

Thank you for taking the time to learn more about stuttering, people who stutter and patient listening.

Discussion and Reflection

You can continue your exploration of having better conversations with people who stutter using some of these questions. You can think about them by yourself or discuss them in small groups. Discussions are richer when you invite people from the group the book is about.

1. Have you ever conversed with a person who stutters? What was that like? Do you remember what you talked about? Did you feel comfortable? Do you have an impression of how the other person felt?
2. What should be the role of the listener in conversation with a person who stutters? Should you try to make them feel comfortable? Compliment them on how well they are doing? Help them with their words? Is it enough to just listen? Or does that seem too passive?
3. Have you ever found you held biases about people who stutter? What did you assume about them? Have your thoughts changed?
4. What positive or negative portrayals of people who stutter have you seen in movies and videos? How do they compare with what you've learned?

5. After reading this book, have you gained understanding of how you should interact with people who stutter? What insights do you have now?
6. Do you think you have ever done something to make someone who stutters feel uncomfortable? What do you wish you could change about that?
7. Do you feel confident that you could respectfully engage with a person who stutters after reading this guide?
8. What are some things that you may or may not do when conversing with someone who stutters?
9. What are some ways to be a patient listener when talking to a person who stutters? Would those ways help you listen better to people who do not stutter?
10. What do you think are the psychological effects of going through bullying as a person who stutters?

Resources

Audible resources

We recommend your explorations include audio and video recordings. Hearing patterns will familiarize you with the many ways people stutter and how they might feel. Listening to a relative, friend or acquaintance who stutters will help you learn their patterns and understand them better.

These are some video channels:

Stuttering Therapy Resources

Youtube.com/@StutteringTherapyResources/featured

SAY: The Stuttering Association for the Young

Say.org/mystuttervideos/

Friends: The National Association of Young People Who Stutter

FriendsWhoStutter.org/videos/

Youtube.com/@OpenStutter

Many individuals have posted videos about stuttering. Look for some that meet your interests. Watch a few and decide which ones are most credible to you, based on what you are learning. Looking for videos on the sites of the associations listed below will give you a start.

You can see a TEDx talk by Sharon Emery on YouTube. Emery wrote the introduction for this guide and helped edit the guide.

Movies

The King's Speech: King George VI's surprise 1936 ascension to the throne of the British Empire. 2010.

Rocket Science: Portrayal of a teen's experiences of living with a stutter. 2007.

My Beautiful Stutter: Documentary explores bullying and community support for five children who stutter. 2020.

Paulie: Friendship between a girl who stutters and a parrot. 1998.

A Family Thing: James Earl Jones as a police officer who stutters. 1996.

The Right Stuff: Shows how astronaut John Glenn's wife, Annie, navigated public appearances with her stutter. 1983.

Blue-Eyed Samurai: Animated series features a kind, strong character who stutters. 2023.

Podcasts

My Stuttering Life

Proud Stutter

StutterTalk

Stuttering Demystified & Beyond

Stuttering Foundation Podcast

Stuttering is Cool

Stutterology

The Stuttering Springboard

Organizations

There are many groups that help people who stutter and allies who want to become better listeners. These are some of the best.

American Board of Stuttering, Cluttering and Fluency Disorders | StutteringSpecialists.org

American Institute for Stuttering | StutteringTreatment.org

The American Speech-Language-Hearing Association | Asha.org

Friends: The National Association of Young People Who Stutter | FriendsWhoStutter.org

International Stuttering Association | ISAStutter.org

Myspeech | MySpeechHub.org

National Stuttering Association | WeStutter.org

SAY: The Stuttering Association for the Young | Say.org

SPACE | SpaceToStutter.org

Stuttering Foundation | StutteringHelp.org

Stuttering Society | StutteringSociety.org

Stuttering Therapy Resources | StutteringTherapyResources.com

Books for adults

Berquez, Ali and Martha Jeffery. *Solution Focused Brief Therapy with Children and Young People Who Stammer and Their Parents: A Practical Guide from the Michael Palin Centre*. Milton Park: Routledge. 2024.

Campbell, Patrick, Christopher Constantino and Sam Simpson. *Stammering Pride and Prejudice: Difference not Defect*. West Sussex: J&R Press. 2020.

Emery, Sharon. *It's Hard Being You: A Primer on Being Happy Anyway*. Traverse City: Mission Point Press. 2022.

Guitar, Barry. *Stuttering: An Integrated Approach to Its Nature and Treatment*, sixth edition. Philadelphia: LWW. 2024.

Gunars K. Neiders and Will Ross. *From Stuttering to Fluency: Manage Your Emotions and Live More Fully*. Independently published on CreateSpace. 2013.

Hayden, James. *Dear World, I Stutter: A Series of Open Letters from a Person Who Stutters*. Independently published on CreateSpace. 2017.

Hendrickson, John. *Life on Delay: Making Peace with a Stutter*. New York City: Knopf. 2023.

Hurwitz, Hanan. *Stuttering: From Shame and Anxiety to Confident Authenticity*. Independently published. 2024.

Mernick, Moe. *The Gift of Stuttering: Confronting Life's Challenges: A Personal Journey*. Nanuet: Feldheim Press. 2016.

Preston, Katherine. *Out With It: How Stuttering Helped Me Find My Voice*. New York City: Atria Books. 2014.

Seay, Taylor. *How to Live with a Stutter: A Survival Guide*. Independently published. 2022.

Silverman, Ellen-Marie. *Relief From Stuttering: Laying the Groundwork to Speak with Greater Ease*. Independently published on CreateSpace. 2013.

Yairi, Ehud and Carol H. Seery. *Stuttering: Foundations and Clinical Applications*, Fifth Edition. San Diego: Plural Publishing, Inc. 2021.

Books for children and young adults

Block, Kim. *Adventures of a Stuttering Superhero: Adventure #1 Interrupt-itis*. Bainbridge Island: Eagle Harbor Books. 2016.

Block, Kim. *Adventures of a Stuttering Superhero: Adventure #2 Melissa Meets Her Stamily*. 2018.

Blodgett, Jack. *Freakin' Iris*. Independently published. 2024.

Boone, Yolanda. *The Adventures of Abigail*. Independently published. 2019.

Charles, Henry. *Stuttering Henry*. Hiztory Bookz. 2022.

Cowley, Ryan. *Worth Waiting For: A Coloring Book for the Stuttering Community*. Independently published. 2025.

Espinosa, Regan. *Santa Stutters Too*. Independently published. 2019.

Heffler, Jason. *Tongue Tied*. 2024.

Hollet, Karen. *Hooray for Aidan*. Hooray Publishing. 2001.

McKinney, John Paul. *An Ode to Cleve*. Miramont Press. 2024.

Rabinowitz, Alan. *A Boy and A Jaguar*. HMH Books. 2014.

Scott, Jordan. *I Talk Like a River*. Neal Porter Books. 2020.

Steinfeld, Steven. *Ettie Stutters: A True Story for Children of All Ages Who Stutter*. Independently published. 2023.

Smith, Lonnie. *Wadey*. Christian Faith. 2020.

Our Story

The 100 Questions and Answers series springs from the idea that good journalism should increase cross-cultural competence and understanding. Most of our guides are created by Michigan State University journalism students.

We use journalistic interviews to surface the simple, everyday questions that people have about each other but might be afraid to ask. We use research and reporting to get the answers and then put them where people can find them, read them and learn about each other.

These cultural competence guides are meant to be conversation starters. We want people to use these guides to get some baseline understanding and to feel comfortable asking more questions. We put a resources section in every guide we make and we arrange community conversations. While the guides can answer questions in private, they are meant to spark discussions.

Making these has taught us that people are not that different from each other. People share more similarities than differences. We all want the same things for ourselves and for our families. We want to be accepted, respected and understood.

Please email your thoughts and suggestions to series editor Joe Grimm at joe.grimm@gmail.com, at the Michigan State University School of Journalism.

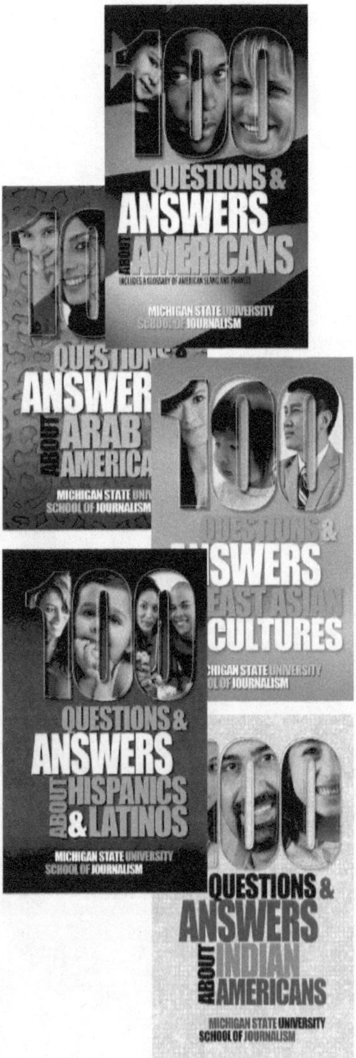

news.jrn.msu.edu/culturalcompetence

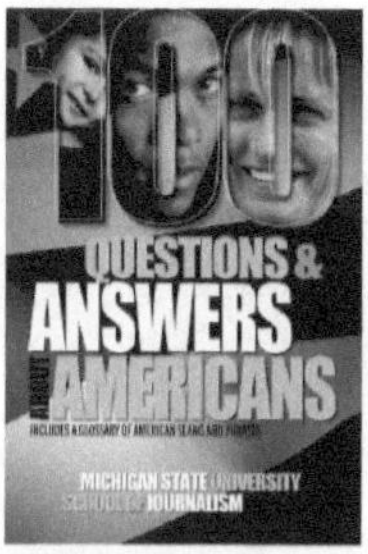

100 Questions and Answers About Americans
Michigan State University School of Journalism, 2013

This guide answers some of the first questions asked by newcomers to the United States. Questions represent dozens of nationalities coming from Africa, Asia, Australia, Europe and North and South America. Good for international students, guests and new immigrants.

ISBN: 978-1-939880-20-8

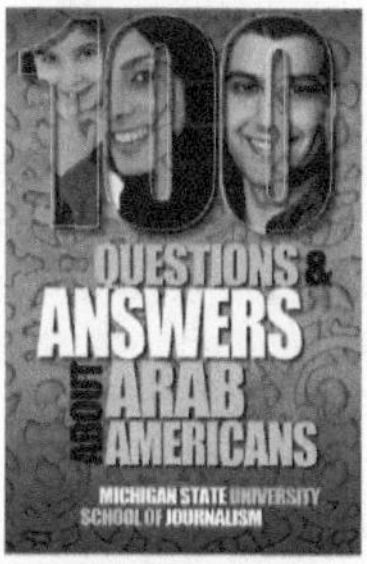

100 Questions and Answers About Arab Americans
Michigan State University School of Journalism, 2014

The terror attacks of Sept. 11, 2001, propelled these Americans into a difficult position where they are victimized twice. The guide addresses stereotypes, bias and misinformation. Key subjects are origins, religion, language and customs. A map shows places of national origin.

ISBN: 978-1-939880-56-7

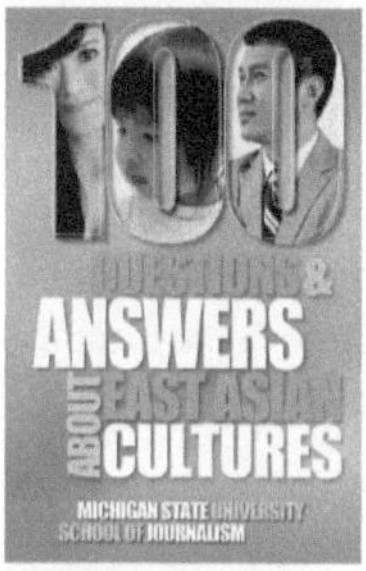

100 Questions and Answers About East Asian Cultures
Michigan State University School of Journalism, 2014

Large university enrollments from Asia prompted this guide as an aid for understanding cultural differences. The focus is on people from China, Japan, Korea and Taiwan and includes Mongolia, Hong Kong and Macau. The guide includes history, language, values, religion, foods and more.

ISBN: 978-939880-50-5

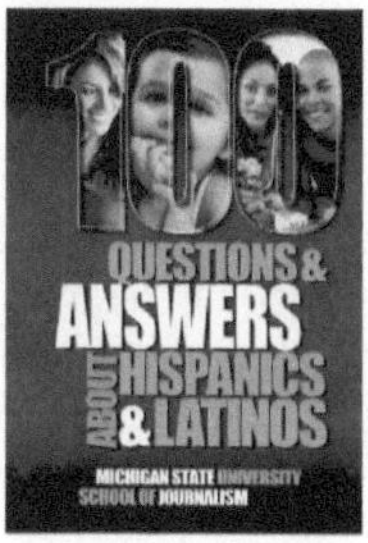

100 Questions and Answers About Hispanics & Latinos
Michigan State University School of Journalism, 2014

This group became the largest ethnic minority in the United States in 2014 and this guide answers many of the basic questions about it. Questions were suggested by Hispanics and Latinos. Includes maps and charts on origin and size of various Hispanic populations.

ISBN: 978-1-939880-44-4

Print and ebooks available on Amazon.com and other retailers.

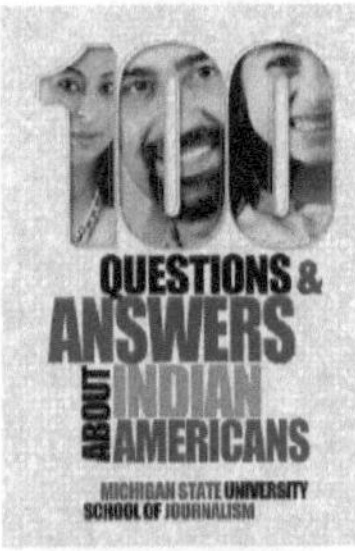

100 Questions and Answers About Indian Americans

Michigan State University School of Journalism, 2013

In answering questions about Indian Americans, this guide also addresses Pakistanis, Bangladeshis and others from South Asia. The guide covers religion, issues of history, colonization and national partitioning, offshoring and immigration, income, education, language and family.

ISBN: 978-1-939880-00-0

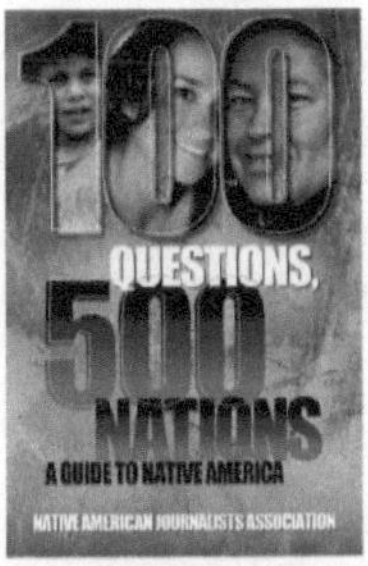

100 Questions, 500 Nations: A Guide to Native America

Michigan State University School of Journalism, 2014

This guide was created in partnership with the Native American Journalists Association. The guide covers tribal sovereignty, treaties and gaming, in addition to answers about population, religion, U.S. policies and politics. The guide includes the list of federally recognized tribes.

ISBN: 978-1-939880-38-3

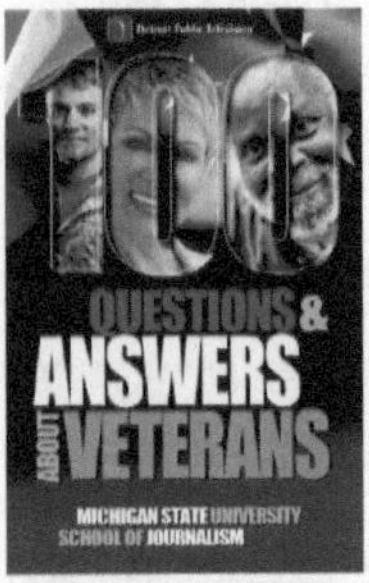

100 Questions and Answers About Veterans

Michigan State University School of Journalism, 2015

This guide treats the more than 20 million U.S. military veterans as a cultural group with distinctive training, experiences and jargon. Graphics depict attitudes, adjustment challenges, rank, income and demographics. Includes six video interviews by Detroit Public Television.

ISBN: 978-1-942011-00-2

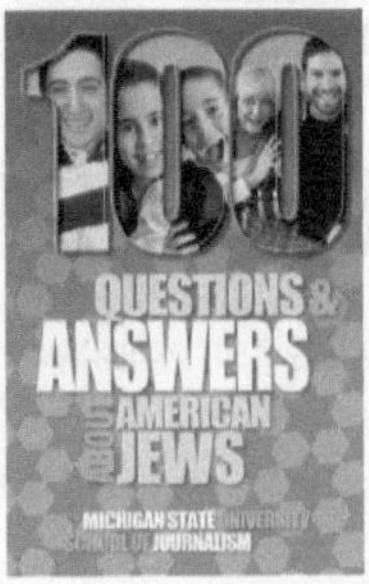

100 Questions and Answers About American Jews

Michigan State University School of Journalism, 2016

We begin by asking and answering what it means to be Jewish in America. The answers to these wide-ranging, base-level questions will ground most people and set them up for meaningful conversations with Jewish acquaintances.

ISBN: 978-1-942011-22-4

news.jrn.msu.edu/culturalcompetence

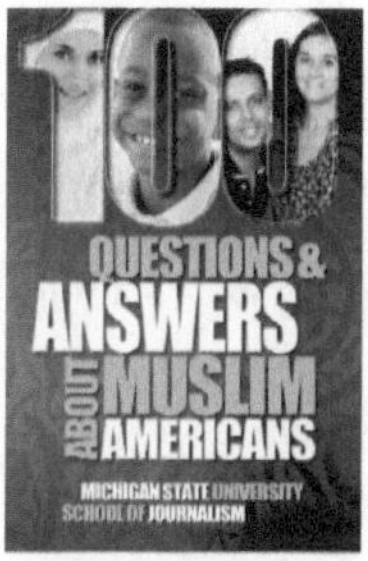

100 Questions and Answers About Muslim Americans
Michigan State University School of Journalism, 2014

This guide was done at a time of rising intolerance in the United States toward Muslims. The guide describes the presence of this religious group around the world and inside the United States. It includes audio on how to pronounce some basic Muslim words.

ISBN: 978-1-939880-79-6

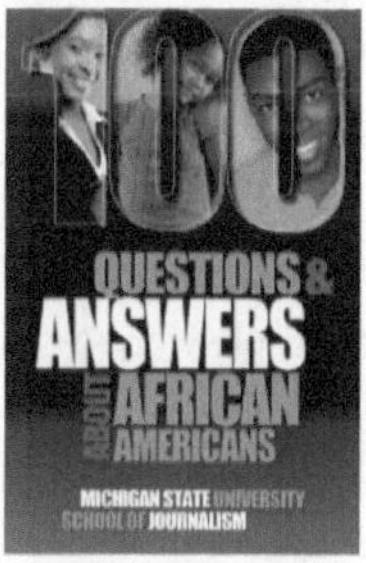

100 Questions and Answers About African Americans
Michigan State University School of Journalism, 2016

Learn about the racial issues that W.E.B. DuBois said in 1900 would be the big challenge for the 20th century. This guide explores Black and African American identity, history, language, contributions and more. Learn more about current issues in American cities and campuses.

ISBN: 978-1-942011-19-4

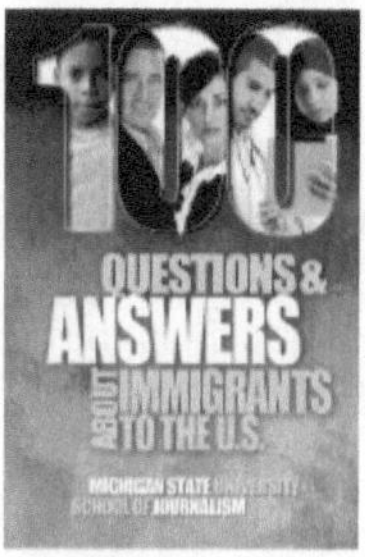

100 Questions and Answers About Immigrants to the U.S.
Michigan State University School of Journalism, 2016

This simple, introductory guide answers 100 of the basic questions people ask about U.S. immigrants and immigration in everyday conversation. It has answers about identity, language, religion, culture, customs, social norms, economics, politics, education, work, families and food.

ISBN: 978-1-934879-63-4

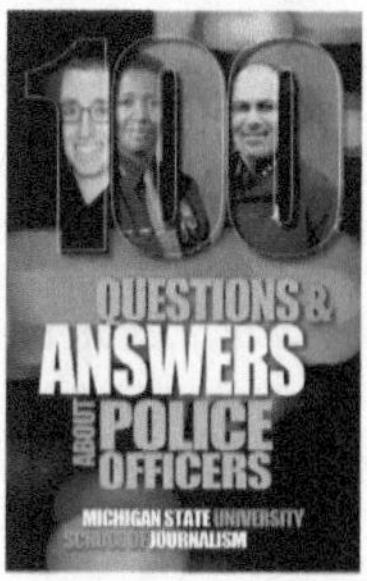

100 Questions and Answers about Police Officers
Michigan State University School of Journalism, 2018

This simple, introductory guide answers 100 of the basic questions people ask about police officers, sheriff's deputies, public safety officers and tribal police. It focuses on policing at the local level, where procedures vary from coast to coast. The guide includes a resource about traffic stops.

ISBN: 978-1-64180-013-6

Print and ebooks available on Amazon.com and other retailers.

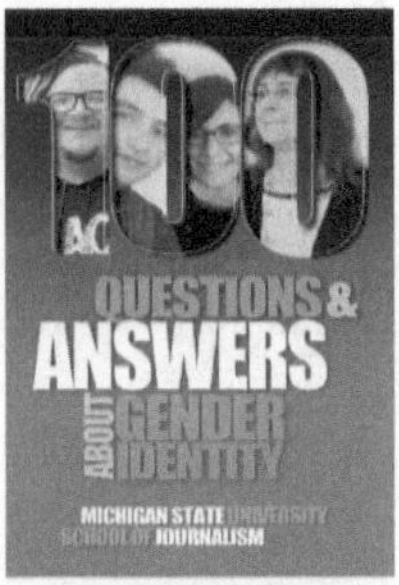

100 Questions and Answers About Gender Identity
Michigan State University School of Journalism, 2017

The guide is written for anyone who wants quick answers to basic, introductory questions about transgender people. It is a starting point people who want to get a fast grounding in the facts.

ISBN: 978-1-641-800-02-0

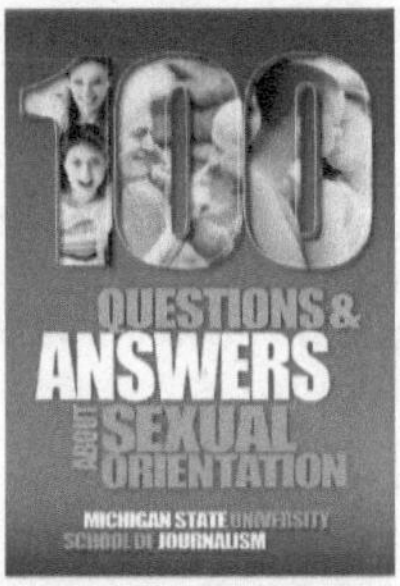

100 Questions and Answers About Sexual Orientation
Michigan State University School of Journalism, 2018

This clear, introductory guide answers 100 of the basic questions people ask about people who are lesbian, gay, bisexual or who have other sexual orientations. The questions come from interviews with people who say these are issues they frequently get asked about or wish people knew more about.

ISBN: 978-1-641-800-27-3

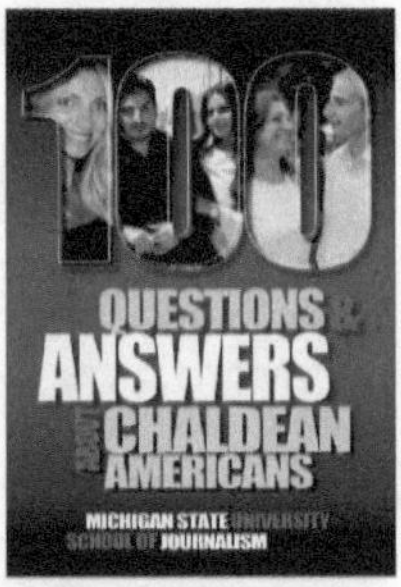

100 Questions and Answers About Chaldean Americans
Michigan State University School of Journalism, 2019

This guide has sections on identity, language, religion, culture, customs, social norms, economics, politics, education, work, families and food. It is written for those who want authoritative answers to basic, questions about this immigrant group from Iraq.

ISBN: 978-1-934-879-63-4

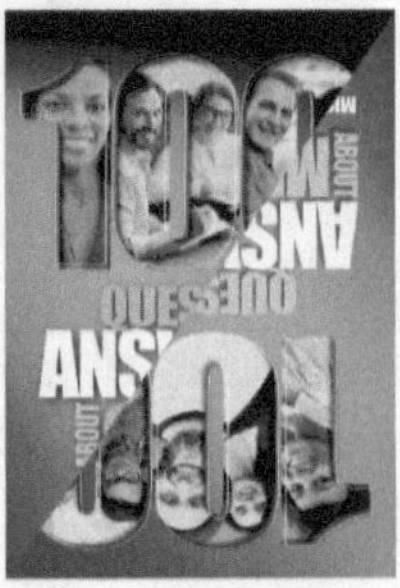

100 Questions and Answers About Gen X Plus
100 Questions and Answers About Millennials
Michigan State University School of Journalism, 2019

This is a double guide in the Bias Busters series. It is written for those who want authoritative answers about these important generations and how we all work together.

ISBN: 978-1-641-800-47-1

news.jrn.msu.edu/culturalcompetence

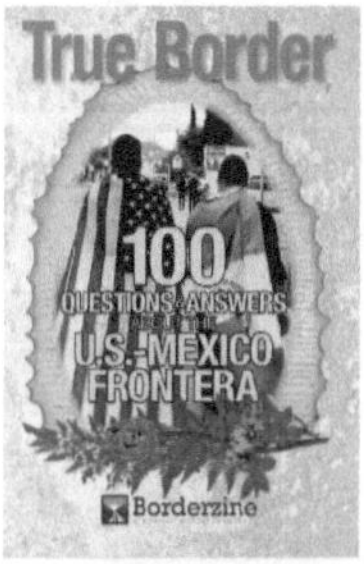

True Border: 100 Questions and Answers About the U.S.-Mexico Frontera
Borderzine: Reporting Across Fronteras, 2020

This guide was developed by the University of Texas/ Borderzine for the Bias Busters cultural competence series. The guide is written for people who want authoritative answers about the U.S.-Mexico border region and get up to speed quickly on this important topic.

ISBN: 978-1-641-800-60-0

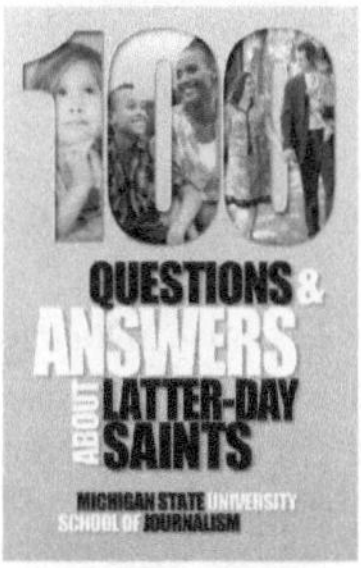

100 Questions and Answers About Latter-day Saints
Michigan State University School of Journalism, 2020

This guide is written for those who want authoritative answers to basic questions about the Latter-day Saints faith. It relies extensively on the Church of Jesus Christ of Latter-day Saints writings and suggests resources for greater depth.

ISBN: 978-1-641-800-90-7

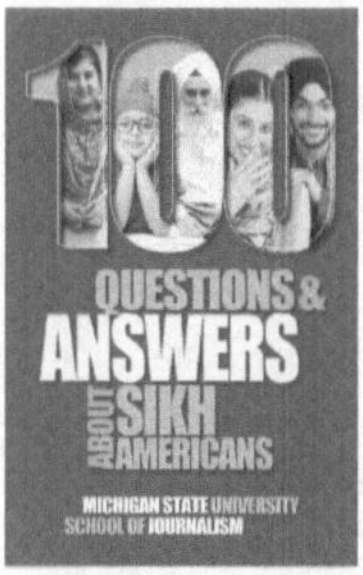

100 Questions and Answers About Sikh Americans
Michigan State University School of Journalism, 2022

Sikhism is the fifth largest religion in the world. It is a young religion, having been founded in 1469. It has been in the United States for almost 150 years, but is still relatively unknown. The questions in this guide were created by interviewing Sikhs.

ISBN: 978-1-641-801-43-0

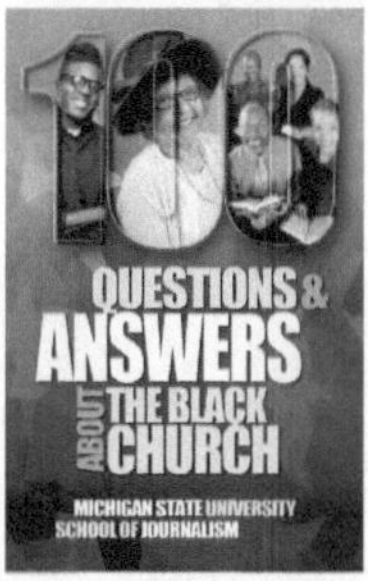

100 Questions and Answers About The Black Church
Michigan State University School of Journalism, 2022

Forged in the furnace of U.S. segregation, the Black Church is the pillar of African American communities across the country. This guide answers the call that TIME magazine raised in a headline, "To understand America, you need to understand the Black Church."

ISBN: 978-1-641-801-55-3

Print and ebooks available on Amazon.com and other retailers.

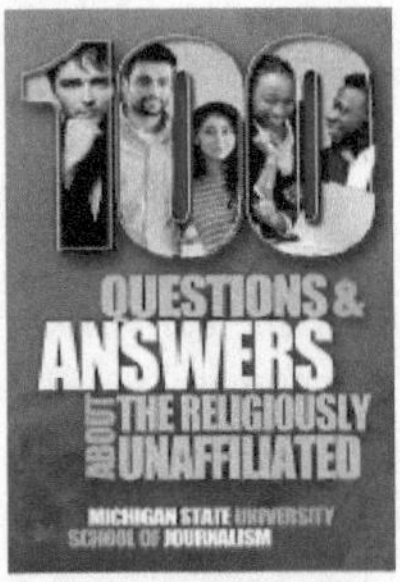

100 Questions and Answers About the Religiously Unaffiliated
Michigan State University School of Journalism, 2024

Sometimes generally referred to as "the nones," agnostics, atheists, humanists, freethinkers, secularists and skeptics compose one of the fastest growing faith categories in the United States. Some people face discrimination as nonbelievers, despite their varied and strong beliefs, values and morals.

ISBN: 978-1-641-801-66-9

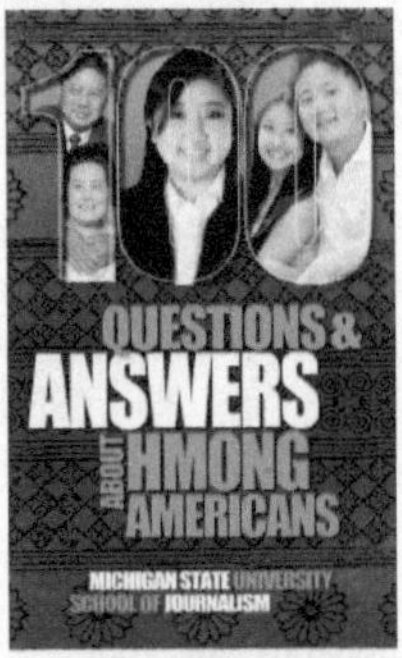

100 Questions and Answers About Hmong Americans
Michigan State University School of Journalism, 2024

In the 50 years since the CIA's secret war against Communists in Vietnam ended, Hmong Americans have built new lives in a country they fought for, even though they did not belong to it. When the United States ended its military involvement in Southeast Asia in 1975, it left its secret allies defenseless among enemies in a hostile land. Neither the Hmong people nor their U.S. hosts were prepared for the change.

ISBN: 978-1-641-801-92-8

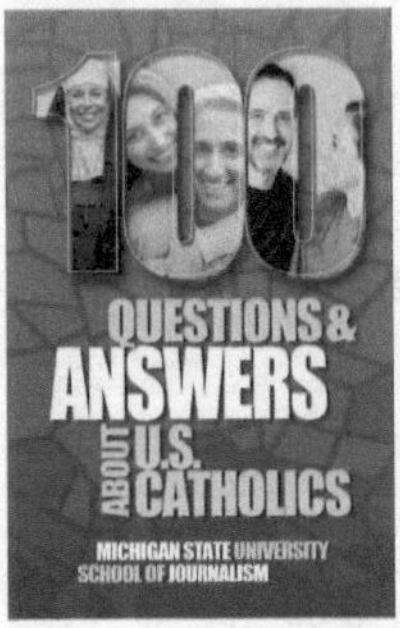

100 Questions and Answers About U.S. Catholics
Michigan State University School of Journalism, 2025

With nearly 70 million Catholics in the U.S., Catholicism touches nearly every corner of American life, from religious holidays and schools to politics and public debates. This book provides respectful answers on everything from Mass to confession, saints, Mary, and the pope to church history, contemporary challenges, and the diversity of American Catholic life today.

ISBN: 978-1-641-802-20-8

news.jrn.msu.edu/culturalcompetence

www.ingramcontent.com/pod-product-compliance
Lightning Source LLC
LaVergne TN
LVHW090331210926
848480LV00004B/1372
9781641802529